I0430102

Table of Contents

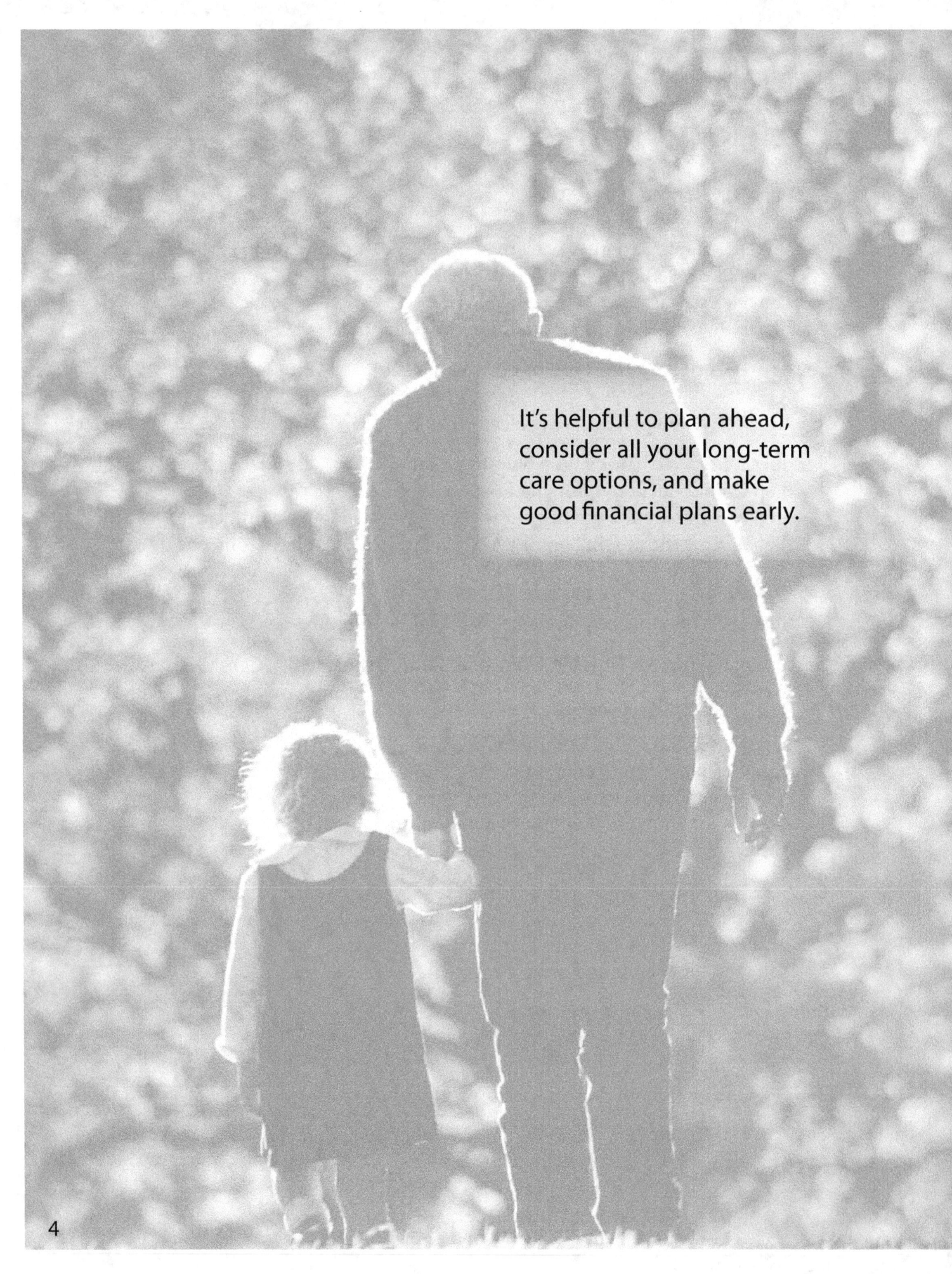

It's helpful to plan ahead, consider all your long-term care options, and make good financial plans early.

Section 1: **Welcome**

The "Guide to Choosing a Nursing Home" is designed to help you make informed decisions about nursing home care, whether you're planning ahead or need to make an unexpected decision. It's helpful to plan ahead, consider all your long-term care options, and make good financial plans early.

Before you get started

You may have other long-term care options, like community services, home care, or assisted living, depending on your needs and resources. It's also possible you may be eligible for home and community-based services covered by Medicaid. Before choosing a nursing home, you can check to see if one of these other options is available to you or if they might help after a nursing home stay. These and other long-term care choices are explained briefly in Section 2.

Not all nursing homes are certified to participate in Medicare or Medicaid. See pages 53–58 for more information on how these programs protect nursing home residents.

If you're helping another person

Helping another person choose a nursing home or make other long-term care choices can be difficult. Your support is important and can help your loved one adjust to getting new services or living in a new place like a nursing home. Be sure to include the person you're helping in decisions whenever possible. Always make decisions with his or her needs and preferences in mind.

If you have Medicare

Medicare generally doesn't cover long-term stays (room and board) in a nursing home. See Section 4 for more information.

See "How to use this booklet" on page 6 to help find the information you need.

How to use this booklet

Is a nursing home your only choice?

Section 2 explains some of the long-term care choices that may be available to you depending on your needs and resources.

Do you need to find a nursing home?

Section 3 outlines steps to find and compare nursing homes and explains where to get answers to your questions. Take the handy tear-out checklist with you when you visit nursing homes.

Once you've chosen a nursing home, what's next?

Section 3 tells you what information you need to have when you make your arrangements to enter a nursing home.

How do you pay for nursing home and other health care?

Section 4 explains how to pay for nursing home and other health care, including personal resources, help from your state, Medicaid, long-term care insurance, and Medicare.

What do you need to know about living in a nursing home?

Section 5 explains how to make the transition from living at home to living in a nursing home easier, how to resolve problems, how your nursing home care is planned, and your resident rights and protections.

Where can you get more information?

Section 6 tells you how to get free Medicare booklets, information about specific health conditions and diseases, and important phone numbers of organizations that can help answer your questions.

What do the words printed in blue mean?

Section 7 explains the words printed in blue throughout this booklet.

Words in blue are defined on pages 67–68.

How can you find specific information in this booklet?

Section 8 is an index (alphabetical list) of what's in this booklet and the page number(s) where you can find specific topics.

Where to get help with your questions

Administration on Aging (AoA)	The AoA is a Federal agency that can give you a list of the long-term care choices in your state including community services. They can also help you find nursing homes. Visit www.aoa.gov or call 1-202-619-0724.
Centers for Medicare & Medicaid Services (CMS)	CMS has free booklets about Medicare and Medicaid coverage, home and community-based services, and other health related topics. See page 59. For information about the location and quality of nursing homes, visit www.medicare.gov/NHCompare. You can also call 1-800-MEDICARE (1-800-633-4227). This is a 24-hour helpline. TTY users should call 1-877-486-2048.
Eldercare Locator	The Eldercare Locator is a nationwide toll-free service to help older adults and their caregivers find local services. Visit www.eldercare.gov or call 1-800-677-1116 (weekdays 9:00 a.m. to 8:00 p.m. EST).
Long-Term Care Ombudsman	A Long-Term Care Ombudsman advocates for residents of nursing homes, board and care homes, and assisted living facilities. See pages 63–65 for the phone number of a Long-Term Care Ombudsman in your state. You may be referred to a local office.
Quality Improvement Organization (QIO)	A QIO is a group of practicing doctors and other health care experts paid by the Federal government to check and improve the care given to people with Medicare. To get the phone number for your QIO, visit www.medicare.gov/contacts or call 1-800-MEDICARE.

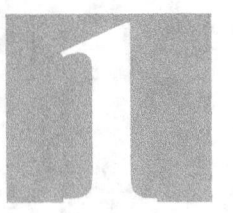

Where to get help with your questions (continued)

State Health Insurance Assistance Program (SHIP)	State Health Insurance Assistance Programs (SHIPs) are state programs. They get money from the Federal government to give free health insurance counseling to people with Medicare. Call them with questions about Medicare, insurance and health plan decisions, and your rights. See pages 63–65 for the phone number for your state.
State Medical Assistance (Medicaid) Office	Your State Medical Assistance (Medicaid) office has information about state programs that help pay health and nursing home costs for people with limited incomes and resources. See pages 63–65 for the phone number for your state.
State Survey Agency	Your State Survey Agency can help with questions or complaints about the quality of care or the quality of life in a nursing home. See pages 63–65 for the phone number for your state.

Words in blue are defined on pages 67–68.

Choosing the Type of Care You Need *2*

American Indian/Alaska Natives can contact their local Indian health provider for more information.

Depending on your needs and resources, you may have other long-term care options available to you. For example, you may be able to get the services and support you need in your own home or in other types of community housing. If you're in a hospital, nursing home, or working with a home health agency (HHA), one of the following can explain your options and help arrange your care: a discharge planner, a social worker, or a representative from a local contact agency for community living.

Each state and community has different services and options. The agencies listed below can give you more information. A list of alternative long-term care choices starts on page 10.

Agencies that can help with long-term care choices

Organization	How they can help
Area Agencies on Aging (AAAs)	AAAs assist adults age 50 and older and their caregivers. To find the AAA in your area, visit **www.eldercare.gov** or call The Eldercare Locator at 1-800-677-1116 weekdays from 9:00 a.m. to 8:00 p.m. (EST).
Aging and Disability Resource Centers (ADRCs)	ADRCs assist people of all incomes and ages. Forty-nine states and some territories have ADRCs. To find out if your area is served by an ADRC, visit **www.adrc-tae.org**.
Centers for Independent Living (CILs)	CILs assist people with disabilities of all incomes and ages. A state-by-state directory of CILs can be found by visiting **www.ncil.org/directory.html**.
State Technology Assistance Project	The State Technology Assistance Project has information on medical equipment and other assistive technology. Visit **www.resna.org** or call the Rehabilitation Engineering and Assistive Technology Society of North America (RESNA) at 1-703-524-6686 to get the contact information for your state.
State Medical Assistance (Medicaid) Office	Your State Medical Assistance (Medicaid) office has information about state programs that help pay health and nursing home costs, as well as services in the community, for people with low incomes and limited resources. See pages 63–65 for the phone number in your state.

Alternative long-term care choices

Listed below are some of the more common kinds of long-term care. Talk to your family, your doctor or other health care provider, or a social worker for help deciding what kind of long-term care you need.

Note: If you have limited income and resources, there may be state programs that help cover some of your costs in some of the long-term care choices mentioned here. Call your State Medical Assistance (Medicaid) office for more information. See pages 63–65 for the phone number for your state.

Community services: A variety of community services might help with your personal care and activities, if these services aren't covered by your health insurance. Some services, like volunteer groups that help with things like shopping or transportation, may be low cost or the group may ask for a voluntary donation. Some services may be available at varied costs, depending on where you live and the services you need. Below is a list of home services and programs that are found in many communities:

- Adult day care
- Meal programs (like Meals-on-Wheels)
- Senior centers
- Friendly visitor programs
- Help with shopping and transportation
- Help with legal questions, bill paying, or other financial matters

For information about community services, call your local Area Agency on Aging, Aging and Disability Resource Center, or Center for Independent Living. See page 9.

Home Care: Depending on your needs, you may be able to get help with your personal care activities (such as laundry, shopping, cooking, and cleaning) at home from family members, friends, or volunteer groups. If you think you need home care, talk to your family to see if they can help with your care or help arrange for other care providers. There are also some home health care agencies that can help with nursing or attendant care in your home. If you're eligible for Medicaid, personal care services in your home may be covered.

Words in blue are defined on pages 67–68.

Remember, Medicare only pays for home health care if you meet certain conditions. To get a free copy of the Medicare booklet "Medicare and Home Health Care," see page 59.

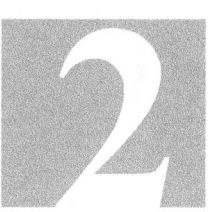
Accessory dwelling units (ADUs): If you or a loved one owns a single-family home, adding an ADU to an existing home may help you keep your independence. An ADU, sometimes called an "in-law apartment," an "accessory apartment," or a "second unit," is a second living space within a home or on a lot. It has a separate living and sleeping area, a place to cook, and a bathroom. Space such as an upper floor, basement, attic, or space over a garage may be turned into an ADU. Family members might be interested in living in an ADU in your home, or, you may want to build a separate living space at a family member's home.

Check with your local zoning office to be sure ADUs are allowed in your area and find out if there are special rules. The cost for an ADU can vary widely depending on how big it is and how much it costs for building materials and workers.

Subsidized senior housing: There are state and Federal programs that help pay for housing for some older people with low to moderate incomes. Some of these housing programs also offer help with meals and other activities, such as housekeeping, shopping, and doing the laundry. Residents usually live in their own apartments within an apartment building. Rent payments are usually a percentage of your income (based on a sliding scale).

Board and care homes: Board and care homes are group living arrangements designed to meet the needs of people who can't live independently but don't need nursing home services. Most board and care homes provide help with some of the activities of daily living, such as bathing, dressing, and using the bathroom. Board and care homes are sometimes called "group homes." Many of these homes aren't paid for by Medicare or Medicaid. The monthly charge is usually a percentage of your income (based on a sliding scale) that covers the cost of rent, meals, and other basic shared services.

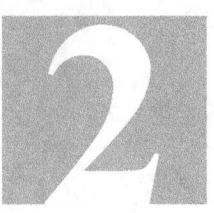

Alternative long-term care choices (continued)

Assisted living facilities: These facilities vary from state to state, but generally they provide help with activities of daily living, such as bathing, dressing, and using the bathroom. They may also help with care most people do themselves, like taking medicine or using eye drops, and additional services, like getting to appointments or preparing meals.

Residents often live in their own room or apartment within a building or group of buildings and have some or all of their meals together. Social and recreational activities are usually provided. Some of these facilities have health services on site.

In most cases, assisted living residents pay a regular monthly rent and pay additional fees for the services they get. Assisted living facilities aren't paid for by Medicare. The term "assisted living" may mean different things in different facilities within the same state. Not all assisted living facilities provide the same services. It's important that you contact the facility and make sure they can meet your needs.

Words in blue are defined on pages 67–68.

Continuing Care Retirement Communities (CCRCs): CCRCs are retirement communities that offer more than one kind of housing and different levels of care. In the same community, there may be individual homes or apartments for residents who still live on their own, an assisted living facility for people who need some help with daily care, and a nursing home for those who require higher levels of care.

Residents move from one level to another based on their individual needs, but usually stay within the CCRC. If you're considering a CCRC, be sure to check the quality information (see pages 16–23) and inspection report (posted in the facility) of its nursing home. Your CCRC contract usually requires you to use the CCRC's nursing home if you need nursing home care. Some CCRCs will only admit people into their nursing home if they are already living in another section of the retirement community.

Many CCRCs generally require a large payment before you move in (called an entry fee) and charge monthly fees. To find out if a CCRC is accredited and get advice on selecting this type of community from the Commission on Accreditation of Rehabilitation Facilities and the Continuing Care Accreditation Commission (CARF-CCAC), visit www.carf.org or call 1-202-587-5001.

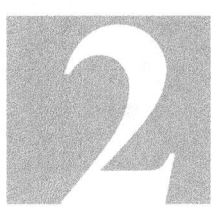

Hospice care: Hospice is a special way of caring for people who are terminally ill (expected to have 6 months or less to live) and for their families. Hospice care includes physical care and counseling. The goal of hospice is to provide comfort for terminal patients and their families, not to cure the illness.

If you qualify for hospice care and you choose hospice, you can get medical and support services, including nursing care, medical social services, doctor services, counseling, homemaker services, and other types of services. As part of hospice care, you will have a team of doctors, nurses, home health aides, social workers, counselors, and trained volunteers to help you and your family cope with your illness. In many cases, you and your family can stay together in your home.

Medicare covers hospice care if you qualify. Depending on your condition, you may get hospice care at home, in a hospice facility, hospital, or nursing home. Medicare doesn't cover room and board if you get general hospice services while you're a resident of a nursing home or a hospice's residential facility. If you're eligible, Medicaid may pay for some services that Medicare doesn't cover, such as personal care assistance at home. Medicare doesn't pay for 24-hour assistance if you get hospice services at home.

Respite care: Some nursing homes and hospice care facilities provide respite care. Respite care is a very short inpatient stay in a nursing home or hospice care facility for a hospice patient so that the usual caregiver can rest. Medicare covers inpatient respite care for up to 5 days if you're getting covered hospice care services. Room and board are covered for inpatient respite care and during short-term hospital stays. If you're eligible, Medicaid will pay for some of these services at home that aren't covered by Medicare.

For more information about Medicare coverage of hospice care and who qualifies, get a free copy of the booklet "Medicare Hospice Benefits." See page 59.

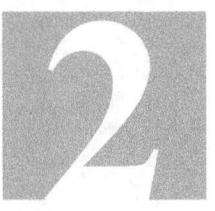

Alternative long-term care choices (continued)

Programs of All-inclusive Care for the Elderly (PACE): PACE is a Medicare and Medicaid Program that manages all of the medical, social, and long-term care services for older people with multiple care needs. It allows people to remain in their homes and maintain their quality of life. PACE is available only in states that have chosen to offer it under Medicaid. The goal of PACE is to help people stay independent and living in their community as long as possible, while getting the high quality care they need. To be eligible for PACE, you must meet the following conditions:

- Be 55 or older
- Live in the service area of a PACE program
- Be certified as eligible for nursing home care by the appropriate state agency
- Be able to live safely in the community

To find out if there is a PACE program in your area, visit www.cms.hhs.gov/PACE or call your State Medical Assistance (Medicaid) office. See pages 63–65.

Home and Community-Based Waiver Programs: If you're already eligible for Medicaid (or, in some states, would be specifically eligible for Medicaid coverage for nursing home services), you may be able to get help with the costs of some home and community-based services, like homemaker services, personal care, and respite care. States have home and community-based waiver programs to help people keep their independence while getting the care they need outside of an inpatient facility.

For more information, call the Area Agency on Aging or the Eldercare Locator (see page 9), or your State Medical Assistance (Medicaid) office. See pages 63–65.

Follow these steps to find the nursing home that meets your needs:

Step 1: Find nursing homes in your area. See below.

Step 2: Compare the quality of nursing homes you're considering. See pages 16–23.

Step 3: Visit the nursing homes you're interested in, or have someone visit for you. See pages 24–36.

Step 4: Choose the nursing home that meets your needs. See pages 37–40.

Step 1: Find out about nursing homes in your area.

Learn about the nursing homes in your area by following these tips:

- Ask people you trust, like your family, friends, neighbors, or clergy if they have had personal experience with nursing homes. They may be able to recommend a nursing home to you.

- Ask your doctor if he or she provides care at any local nursing homes. If so, ask which nursing homes he or she visits so you may continue to see your doctor while you're in the nursing home.

- Visit the Eldercare Locator at www.eldercare.gov or call 1-800-677-1116 for more information on long-term care choices in your area. You can also contact your local Agency on Aging or Senior & Community Activity Center.

- If you're in the hospital, ask your nurse about discharge planning as early in your hospital stay as possible. The hospital's staff should be able to help you find a nursing home that meets your needs and help with your transfer before your hospital discharge.

- If you or someone you know has access to the Internet, visit Medicare's Nursing Home Compare at www.medicare.gov/NHCompare to help you find and compare nursing homes in your area. You can search by nursing home name, city, county, state, or ZIP code. Your local library may be able to help you find the information on Nursing Home Compare if you don't have access to the Internet. You can also call 1-800-MEDICARE (1-800-633-4227) to ask for a printed copy of Nursing Home Comparison be mailed to you. TTY users should call 1-877-486-2048.

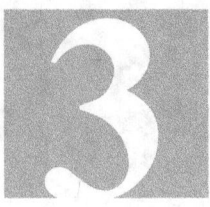

Step 2: Compare the quality of the nursing homes you're considering.

It's important to compare the care that nursing homes give in order to find the nursing home that meets your needs. If you or someone you know has Internet access, you can compare nursing home quality on Nursing Home Compare at www.medicare.gov/NHCompare. Nursing Home Compare has information about certified Medicare and Medicaid nursing homes. Maps and directions to nursing homes are also available.

Words in blue are defined on pages 67–68.

On Nursing Home Compare, you can compare the nursing homes you're considering by the following:

- The Five Star Quality Rating
- Detailed information on health inspections
- Nursing home staffing
- Quality measures
- Fire safety inspections

Note: Information on Nursing Home Compare isn't an endorsement or advertisement for any nursing home. You may want to use a variety of resources when choosing a nursing home. Don't rely only on the nursing home's star rating to make a final decision. Visit the nursing homes you're considering, if possible, or have someone visit for you.

These ratings are combined for an overall quality rating. Information about fire safety inspections is included on Nursing Home Compare to give you more information about a nursing home's overall quality.

Five Star Quality Rating System

The Five Star Quality Rating System on Nursing Home Compare is designed to:

- Give an overall picture of nursing homes so you can see meaningful differences between high- and low-performing nursing homes
- Give you easy-to-use information to help you choose a nursing home for yourself or others
- Give you information about the care in nursing homes where you or a family member may already live
- Guide you in talking to nursing home staff about the quality of care

Health inspections

To be a certified provider under Medicare and/or Medicaid, nursing homes have to meet more than 150 regulations that Congress has set to protect nursing home residents. These regulations cover a wide range of topics, from protecting residents from physical or mental abuse and inadequate care to the safe storage and preparation of food.

Note: Not all nursing homes are certified to participate in Medicare or Medicaid. Remember to ask whether the nursing home you're visiting participates in one or both of these programs.

The Centers for Medicare & Medicaid Services (CMS) has contracts with state governments to do health and fire safety inspections of these certified nursing homes and investigate complaints about nursing home care. The health inspection team consists of trained surveyors, including at least one registered nurse. These inspections take place, on average, about once a year, but may be done more often if the nursing home is performing poorly.

Using the Federal regulations, the state inspection team looks at many aspects of life in the nursing home including the following:

- The residents' care and how care is given by the staff
- How the staff talks to and treats the residents
- The activities and daily life of the residents
- The condition of resident rooms and the cleanliness, sanitation, and maintenance of the nursing home

In order to do this, the surveyors review the residents' clinical records, interview residents about their life in the nursing home, interview family members about the care their loved one gets, and interview staff, such as nursing aides, activities staff, dietary staff, and administrative staff.

You can use health survey information on Nursing Home Compare to see what health and safety regulations a nursing home failed to meet during recent health surveys.

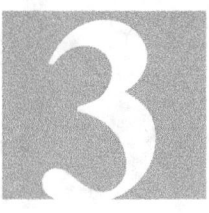

Step 2: Compare the quality of the nursing homes you're considering (continued).

Nursing home staffing

Federal law requires all Medicare and/or Medicaid-certified nursing homes provide enough staff to provide care for each resident based on their needs, but there is no current Federal standard for the best staffing levels.

The Medicare and/or Medicaid-certified nursing home must have at least one licensed Registered Nurse (RN) for at least 8 hours per day, 7 days a week, and other nursing staff, such as an RN or Licensed Practical Nurse/Licensed Vocational Nurse (LPN/LVN), on duty 24 hours per day. Certain states may have additional staffing requirements. Certified Nursing Assistants (CNAs) are generally on staff 24 hours per day. They work under the supervision of a licensed nurse to help residents with daily activities, such as eating, bathing, and dressing. All CNAs must complete a competency evaluation program or a nurse assistant training within 4 months of their permanent employment. They must also take continuing education training each year.

Some nursing homes may require more staff due to the specific conditions of their residents, along with other factors such as whether the nursing home has special care units. Look at the Nursing Home Checklist on pages 31–36 for questions or observations about staffing that can help you evaluate the nursing homes you visit.

The staffing numbers on Nursing Home Compare are based on information reported by the nursing home for a 2-week period prior to the time of the state inspection. This staffing information is checked only for unusual reporting issues. It's important for you to check out the staffing when you're visiting the nursing home.

Quality measures

Nursing homes regularly collect certain information about the health, physical functioning, mental status, and general well-being of residents, using a screening tool called the "Minimum Data Set" (or "MDS"). Nursing homes are required to complete the MDS on each nursing home resident on admission and whenever the resident's condition changes. The information from the MDS is collected electronically by CMS for each person living in a certified nursing home in the country. CMS uses some of the MDS information to measure the quality of certain aspects of nursing home care, such as whether residents have developed a pressure ulcer, are in pain, or are losing weight. These measures are called "quality measures."

The quality measures on Nursing Home Compare are based on the best research currently available. As this research continues, scientists will keep improving the quality measures used on Nursing Home Compare. However, CMS doesn't set benchmarks, thresholds, guidelines, or standards of care for Medicare and/or Medicaid-certified nursing homes. The quality measures are based on care provided to the population of residents in a facility, not to any individual resident. The quality measures were chosen because they show important ways nursing homes differ from one another.

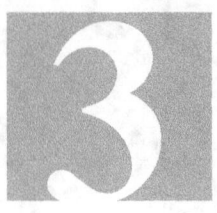

Step 2: Compare the quality of the nursing homes you're considering (continued).

Fire safety inspections

Fire safety specialists inspect nursing homes to see if they meet Life Safety Code (LSC) standards. The LSC is a set of fire protection requirements designed to provide a reasonable degree of safety from fire.

The fire safety inspection covers a wide range of aspects of fire protection, including construction, protection, and operational features designed to provide safety from fire, smoke, and panic. When an inspection team finds that a nursing home doesn't meet a specific LSC regulation, it issues a deficiency citation.

You can use the information about fire safety inspections on Nursing Home Compare to see what fire safety standards a nursing home failed to meet, the level of potential harm, the number of residents this affected, and the date of correction.

Important: While comparing nursing homes, you may want to contact the nursing home to find out about their sprinkler system.

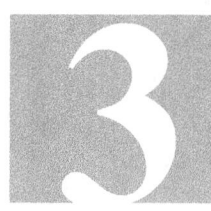

Other ways to find out about nursing home quality

- Call your Long-Term Care Ombudsman. See pages 63–65. The Ombudsman program helps nursing home residents solve problems by acting on their behalf. Long-Term Care Ombudsmen:

  — Visit nursing homes and speak with residents throughout the year to make sure residents' rights are protected

  — Work to solve problems with your nursing home care, including financial issues

  — Discuss general information about nursing homes and nursing home care

  — Help you compare a nursing home's strengths and weaknesses

  — Answer questions, such as how many complaints they have gotten about a specific nursing home, what kind of complaints they were, and if the issues were resolved in a timely manner

- Call the local office of consumer affairs for your state (look in the blue pages in the phone book). Ask if they have written information on the quality of care given in local nursing homes.

- Call your state health department or state licensing agency (look in the blue pages in the phone book). Ask if they have written information on the quality of care given in local nursing homes.

Words in blue are defined on pages 67–68.

Step 2: Compare the quality of the nursing homes you're considering (continued).

Other ways to find out about nursing home quality (continued)

Resident-directed care and the culture change movement

There is a growing, nationwide movement among many nursing homes to change the nursing home culture from rigid institutional living to living in a setting more like a home. Nursing homes involved in this "culture change" practice resident-directed or resident-centered care which promotes greater resident choice over their schedules (such as getting up, going to sleep, method and timing of bathing) and their activities. It also involves changes to the building environment to enhance the residents' quality of life.

Many homes involved in this culture change have "households" within their former living units, which include small groups of residents (usually less than 20). This group of residents has the same staff assigned to them and has activities and meals together. Each household has a kitchen, dining room, and living room space.

A small number of nursing homes have sets of free-standing houses on-campus that contain approximately 10–12 residents, each with private rooms and settings much more like that of a large, private home. Other homes have remodeled their buildings to include more private rooms and a new style of "privacy-enhanced, shared rooms" which have a partial wall separating each resident's half of a room.

Whether in small houses or households in larger buildings, assigning the same staff on most days lets the nursing home staff and residents form close relationships. This way, staff can more fully meet residents' needs and preferences and help them reach their highest level of well-being and functioning. Some homes have been unable to remodel into households but have embraced the principles of culture change by assigning the same staff to residents and giving residents much greater resident choice in their daily lives.

Often culture changing homes have resident dogs and cats and some let a resident bring in his or her own pet (with staff or volunteers assisting the resident with pet care). Other homes have connections to a day care setting in which elders and children interact regularly.

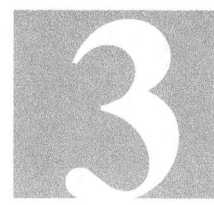

Resident-directed care and the culture change movement (continued)

For more information on resident-directed care and the culture change movement, look at Web sites for culture change, such as Pioneer Network, a non-profit organization at www.pioneernetwork.net.

Facility quality assurance and quality improvement campaigns

All nursing homes are required to have a committee to review any issues of concern with the quality of care and quality of life of residents. The committees must also address and correct these issues on an ongoing basis using principles of continuous quality improvement. Also, many nursing homes are currently participating in public quality improvement campaigns. Knowing that a nursing home participates in one may be a good indicator of the home's commitment to improving quality. One example of a quality improvement campaign is the Advancing Excellence in America's Nursing Homes, a coalition-based campaign to improve the quality of life for residents and staff in America's nursing homes. This particular campaign includes long-term care providers, caregivers, medical and quality improvement experts, consumers, government agencies, and other quality-focused organizations. For more information, visit www.nhqualitycampaign.org.

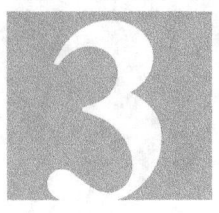

Step 3: Visit the nursing homes you're interested in, or have someone visit for you.

Before you visit any nursing homes, consider what's important to you and think about the following questions:

Quality of life

- Will I be treated in a respectful way?

- Can I participate in social, recreational, religious, or cultural activities that are important to me? Can I decide when I want to participate?

- Do I get to choose what time to get up, go to sleep, or bathe?

- Can I get food and drinks that I like at any time? What if I don't like the food that is served?

- Can I have visitors at any time?

- Is transportation provided to community activities?

- Can I bring my pet or can my pet visit?

- Can I decorate my living space any way I want?

- Will I have privacy when I have visitors or personal care services?

- Would I be able to leave the facility for a few hours or days if I choose to do so?

3

Quality of care

- What's a plan of care and what does it look like?
- Who makes the plan of care and how do they know what I want, need, or what should be in the plan?
- Will I be included in planning my care?
- Will my interests and preferences be included in the care plan?
- Will I be able to change the plan if I feel there is a need?
- Will I be able to choose which of my family members or friends will be involved in the planning process?
- Will I get a copy of my care plan?
- Is there enough staff to give me the care I need?
- Who are the doctors that will care for me? Can I still see my personal doctors? Who will help me arrange transportation if I choose to continue to see my personal doctors and they don't visit the nursing home?
- Who will give me the care I need?
- If a resident has a problem with confusion and wanders, how does the staff handle this type of behavior in the facility to protect the resident?
- Does the nursing home's inspection report show quality of care problems (deficiencies)?
- What did the quality information on "Nursing Home Compare" at www.medicare.gov/NHCompare show about how well this nursing home cares for its residents?

Location

- Is the nursing home close to my family and friends so they can visit often?

Availability

- Is a bed available now or can I add my name to a waiting list?

Note: Nursing homes don't have to accept all applicants, but they must comply with local, state, and Federal civil rights laws that prohibit discrimination.

Step 3: Visit the nursing homes you're interested in, or have someone visit for you (continued).

Staffing

- Will I have the same staff people take care of me from day to day or do they change?

- Does the nursing home post required information about the number of licensed and unlicensed nursing staff? Are they willing to show me if I ask to see it?

- How many residents is a Certified Nursing Assistant (CNA) assigned to work with during each shift (day and night) and during meals?

- If I have a medical need, will the staff contact my doctor for me?

- What type of therapy is available at this facility? Is therapy staff available?

- Is there a social worker available? Can I meet him or her?

Religious and Cultural Preferences

- Does the nursing home offer the religious or cultural support I need? If not, what type of arrangements will they provide to meet my needs?

- Do they provide special diet options that my faith practice may require?

Language

- Is my primary language spoken by staff that will work directly with me and fellow residents?

- If not, is an interpreter available or another system in place to help me communicate my needs?

Policies

- Are there resident policies I must follow?

- Will I get a written copy of these policies?

Note: Policies are rules that all residents must follow. For example, smoking may not be allowed in the nursing home.

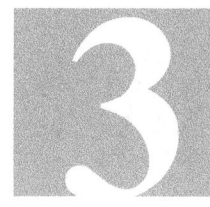

Security

- Does the nursing home provide a safe environment?
- Will my personal belongings be secure in my room?
- Is the nursing home locked at night?

Preventive care

- Does the nursing home make sure residents get preventive care to help keep them healthy? Are specialists, like eye doctors, ear doctors, dentists, and podiatrists, available to see residents on a regular basis? Does the facility help make arrangement to see these specialists?
- Does the nursing home have a screening program for vaccinations, such as flu (influenza) and pneumonia?

Hospitals

- Does the nursing home have an arrangement with a nearby hospital for emergencies?
- Can my doctor care for me at that hospital?

Licensing

- Are the nursing home and current administrator licensed in my state?

Note: This means nursing homes have met certain standards set by a state or local government agency.

Certification (certified)

- Is the nursing home Medicare and/or Medicaid-certified?

Note: "Certified" means the nursing home meets Medicare and/or Medicaid regulations and the nursing home has passed an inspection survey done by the State Survey Agency. If they're certified, make sure they haven't recently lost their certification or are about to lose their certification. Also, some nursing homes may only have a certain part of their building for Medicare or Medicaid residents.

Words in blue are defined on pages 67–68.

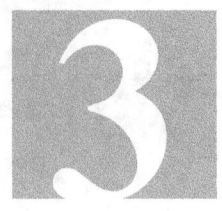

Step 3: Visit the nursing homes you're interested in, or have someone visit for you (continued).

Services

- What services does the nursing home provide? Does the nursing home have the services I need?

Charges and fees

- Will the nursing home tell me in writing about their services, charges, and fees before I move into the home.

  Note: Medicare and/or Medicaid-certified nursing homes must tell you this information in writing. Get a copy of the fee schedule to find out which services are available, which are included in your monthly fee, and which services cost extra. Then, compare nursing home costs.

- Is there a basic fee for room, meals, and personal care?

- Are there extra charges for other services, such as beauty shop services?

Health inspection and fire safety inspection reports

- Does the nursing home have the most recent health and fire inspection reports for me to look at?

  Note: Ask the staff to provide these reports. They tell you how well the nursing home meets Federal health and safety regulations. The nursing home must have the report of the most recent state or Federal survey of the facility available for you to look at.

Resident, family, and staff satisfaction

- Can I talk to staff, residents, and family members of residents? Will I be able to ask them if they're satisfied with the nursing home and its services?

  Note: Any resident or family member of a resident has the right to refuse to talk to you. However, staff should be able to visit with you if they're not involved in care or service duties at the time.

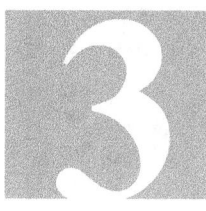

Visit the nursing homes

After you consider what's important to you in a nursing home, visit the nursing homes. It's best to visit the nursing homes that interest you before you make a final decision on which one meets your needs.

A visit gives you the chance to see the residents, staff, and the nursing home setting. It also allows you to ask questions of the nursing home staff and talk with residents and their family members.

If you can't visit the nursing home yourself, you may want to get a family member or friend to visit for you. If a family member or friend can't visit for you, you can call for information. However, a visit can help you see the quality of care and life of the actual residents.

Important things to know when visiting a nursing home:

- Before you go, call and make an appointment to meet with someone on staff. You're also encouraged to visit the nursing home at other times without an appointment. If a nursing home doesn't offer a "drop-in" policy, this is another issue to think about when making your final decision.

- Don't be afraid to ask questions.

- Ask the staff to explain anything you see and hear that you don't understand. For example, if you hear a person calling out, it may be because they're confused, not because they're being hurt or neglected.

- Ask who to call if you have further questions and write down the name and phone number.

- If a resident or a resident's family wishes, you may talk to them about the care and their experience.

- Don't go into resident rooms or care areas without asking the resident and nursing home staff first. Residents have a right to privacy and can refuse to allow you to come into their rooms.

- After your visit, write down any questions you still have about the nursing home or how the nursing home will meet your needs.

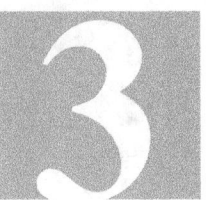

The Nursing Home Checklist

Use the Nursing Home Checklist when you visit a nursing home.

Take a copy of the Nursing Home Checklist (see pages 30–36) when you visit to ask questions about resident life, nursing home living spaces, staff, residents' rooms, hallways, stairs, lounges, bathrooms, menus and food, activities, safety, and care.

Use a new checklist for each nursing home you visit. You can photocopy the checklist or print additional copies available at www.medicare.gov/NHCompare.

Name of Nursing Home: _____

Address: _____

Phone Number: _____

Date of Visit: _____

Basic Information	Yes	No	Comment
Is the nursing home Medicare-certified?			
Is the nursing home Medicaid-certified?			
Does the nursing home have the level of care I need?			
Does the nursing home have a bed available?			
Does the nursing home offer specialized services, such as a special unit for care for a resident with dementia, ventilator care, or rehabilitation services?			
Is the nursing home located close enough for friends and family to visit?			

The Nursing Home Checklist

Resident Appearance	Yes	No	Comment
Are the residents clean, well groomed, and appropriately dressed for the season or time of day?			

Nursing Home Living Spaces	Yes	No	Comment
Is the nursing home free from overwhelming unpleasant odors?			
Does the nursing home appear clean and well kept?			
Is the temperature in the nursing home comfortable for residents?			
Does the nursing home have good lighting?			
Are the noise levels in the dining room and other common areas comfortable?			
Is smoking allowed? If so, is it restricted to certain areas of the nursing home?			
Are the furnishings sturdy, yet comfortable and attractive?			

3

The Nursing Home Checklist

Staff	Yes	No	Comment
Does the relationship between the staff and residents appear to be warm, polite, and respectful?			
Does the staff wear name tags?			
Does the staff knock on the door before entering a resident's room? Do they refer to residents by name?			
Does the nursing home offer a training and continuing education program for all staff?			
Does the nursing home check to make sure they don't hire staff members who have been found guilty of abuse, neglect or mistreatment of residents; or have a finding of abuse, neglect, or mistreatment of residents in the state nurse aid registry?			
Is there a licensed nursing staff 24 hours a day, including a Registered Nurse (RN) present at least 8 hours per day, 7 days a week?			
Will a team of nurses and Certified Nursing Assistants (CNAs) work with me to meet my needs?			
Do CNAs help plan the care of residents?			
Is there a person on staff that will be assigned to meet my social service needs?			
If I have a medical need, will the staff contact my doctor for me?			
Has there been a turnover in administration staff, such as the administrator or director of nurses, in the past year?			

The Nursing Home Checklist

Residents' Rooms	Yes	No	Comment
Can residents have personal belongings and furniture in their rooms?			
Does each resident have storage space (closet and drawers) in his or her room?			
Does each resident have a window in his or her bedroom?			
Do residents have access to a personal phone and television?			
Do residents have a choice of roommates?			
Are there policies and procedures to protect residents' possessions, including lockable cabinets and closets?			

Hallway, Stairs, Lounges, and Bathrooms	Yes	No	Comment
Are exits clearly marked?			
Are there quiet areas where residents can visit with friends and family?			
Does the nursing home have smoke detectors and sprinklers?			
Are all common areas, resident rooms, and doorways designed for wheelchair use?			
Are handrails and grab bars appropriately placed in the hallways and bathrooms?			

3

The Nursing Home Checklist

Menus and Food	Yes	No	Comment
Do residents have a choice of food items at each meal? (Ask if your favorite foods are served.)			
Can the nursing home provide for special dietary needs (like low-salt or no-sugar-added diets)?			
Are nutritious snacks available upon request?			
Does the staff help residents eat and drink at mealtimes if help is needed?			

Activities	Yes	No	Comment
Can residents, including those who are unable to leave their rooms, choose to take part in a variety of activities?			
Do residents have a role in planning or choosing activities that are available?			
Does the nursing home have outdoor areas for resident use? Is the staff available to help residents go outside?			
Does the nursing home have an active volunteer program?			

The Nursing Home Checklist

Safety and Care	Yes	No	Comment
Does the nursing home have an emergency evacuation plan and hold regular fire drills (bed-bound residents included)?			
Do residents get preventive care, like a yearly flu shot, to help keep them healthy? Does the facility assist in arranging hearing screenings or vision tests?			
Can residents still see their personal doctors? Does the facility help in arranging transportation for this purpose?			
Does the nursing home have an arrangement with a nearby hospital for emergencies?			
Are care plan meetings held with residents and family members at times that are convenient and flexible whenever possible?			
Has the nursing home corrected all deficiencies (failure to meet one or more state or Federal requirements) on its last state inspection report?			

3

The Nursing Home Checklist

Go to a resident council or family council meeting

While you're visiting the nursing home, ask a member of the resident council if you can attend a resident council or family council meeting. These councils are usually organized and managed by the residents or the residents' families to address concerns and improve the quality of care and life for the resident.

If you're able to go to a meeting, ask a council member the following questions and take notes:

- What improvements were made to the quality of life for residents in the last year? _____

- What are the plans for future improvements? _____

- How has the nursing home responded to recommendations for improvement? _____

- Who does the council report to? _____

- How does membership on the council work? _____

- Who sets the agendas for meetings? _____

- How are decisions made (for example, by voting, consensus, or one person makes them)? _____

Visit again

It's a good idea to visit the nursing home a second time. It's best to visit a nursing home on a different day of the week and at a different time of day than your initial visit. Staffing can be different at different times of the day and on weekends.

Notes on second visit: _____

_____

_____

_____

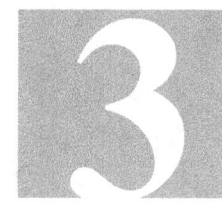

Step 4: Choose the nursing home that meets your needs.

When you have all the information about the nursing homes you're interested in, talk with people who understand your personal and health care needs. This might include your family, friends, doctor, clergy, spiritual advisor, hospital discharge planner, or social worker.

If you find more than one nursing home you like with a bed available, use all the information you get to compare them. Trust your senses. If you didn't like what you saw on a visit, for example, if the facility wasn't clean or if you weren't comfortable talking to the nursing home staff, you may want to choose another nursing home. If you felt that the residents were treated well, the facility was clean, and the staff was helpful, you might feel better about choosing that nursing home.

If you're helping someone, keep the person you're helping involved in making the decision as much as possible. People who are involved from the beginning are better prepared when they move into a nursing home. If the person you're helping isn't alert or able to communicate well, keep his or her values and preferences in mind.

Important: If you visit a nursing home that you don't like, look at other options, if available. Quality care is important. If you're in a hospital, talk to the hospital discharge planner or your doctor before you decide not to go to a nursing home that has an available bed. They may be able to help you find a more suitable nursing home or arrange for other care, such as short-term homecare, until a bed is available at another nursing home you choose. However, you may be responsible for paying the bill for any additional days you stay in the hospital.

Step 4: Choose the nursing home that meets your needs (continued).

Moving is difficult. However, an extra move may be better for you than choosing to stay at a facility that isn't right for you. Be sure to explain to your doctor or discharge planner why you aren't happy with a facility that they may be recommending.

Once in the nursing home, if you find that you don't like the nursing home you chose, you can move to another facility with an available bed. The nursing home you leave may require that you let them know ahead of time that you're planning to leave. Talk to the nursing home staff about their rules for leaving. If you don't follow the rules for leaving, you may have to pay extra fees.

What information is needed?

After you choose a nursing home, you will need to make the arrangements for admission. When you contact the nursing home office, it's helpful to have the following information ready:

Payment information for nursing home office staff

Insurance information: Provide information about any health care coverage and long-term care insurance you have that pays for nursing home care, health care, or both. This includes the name of the insurance company and the policy number.

Note: If nursing home care will be covered by Medicare or Medicaid, the nursing home can't require you to pay a cash deposit. They may ask that you pay your Medicare coinsurance amounts and other charges you would normally have to pay. It's best to pay these charges when they're billed, not in advance. You may have to pay a cash deposit before you're admitted to a nursing home if your care **won't** be covered by either Medicare or Medicaid.

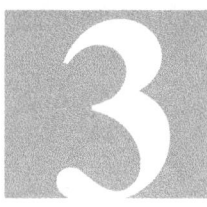

Information for nursing home staff

- **Information on your medical history:** Your doctor may give the staff some of this information. This includes a list of any current or past health problems, any past surgeries or treatments, any shots you've had, and allergies you have to food or medicine.

- **Information on your current health status:** Your doctor should give the staff this information, including a list of your current health problems, recent diagnostic test results, and information about any activities of daily living that might be difficult for you to do by yourself.

- **A list of your current medicines:** Include the dose, how often you take it, and why you take it.

- **A list of all your health care providers:** Include names, addresses, and phone numbers.

- **A list of family members to call in case of an emergency:** Include names, addresses, and phone numbers.

Health care advance directives

You may be asked if you have a health care advance directive. A health care advance directive is a written document that says how you want medical decisions to be made if you become unable to make decisions for yourself. There are two common types of health care advance directives:

- **A Living Will:** A written legal document that shows what type of treatments you want or don't want in case you can't speak for yourself. Usually, this document only comes into effect if you're unconscious and can't speak for yourself. A Living Will tells others what medical care or treatment you want, such as whether you want life support, like a respirator.

- **A durable power of attorney for health care:** A legal document that names someone else to make health care decisions for you. This is helpful if you become unable to make your own decisions.

If you don't have a health care advance directive and need help preparing one, or need more information, talk to a social worker, discharge planner, your doctor, or the nursing home staff. You can call your local Area Agency on Aging to find out if your state has any legal services that help with preparing these forms. See page 9 for their phone number.

Step 4: Choose the nursing home that meets your needs (continued).

Personal needs accounts

You may want to open an account managed by the nursing home, although the nursing home may not require you to. You can deposit money into the account for personal use. Check with the nursing home to see how they manage these accounts. You may only have access to the account at certain times. See pages 55–56 for information about your resident rights and protections regarding money.

Information about Medicare and Medicaid benefits

For people seeking admission to a nursing home, the nursing home must provide (orally and in writing) and prominently display written information about how to apply for and use Medicare and Medicaid benefits. They must also provide information on how to get refunds for previous payments covered by such benefits.

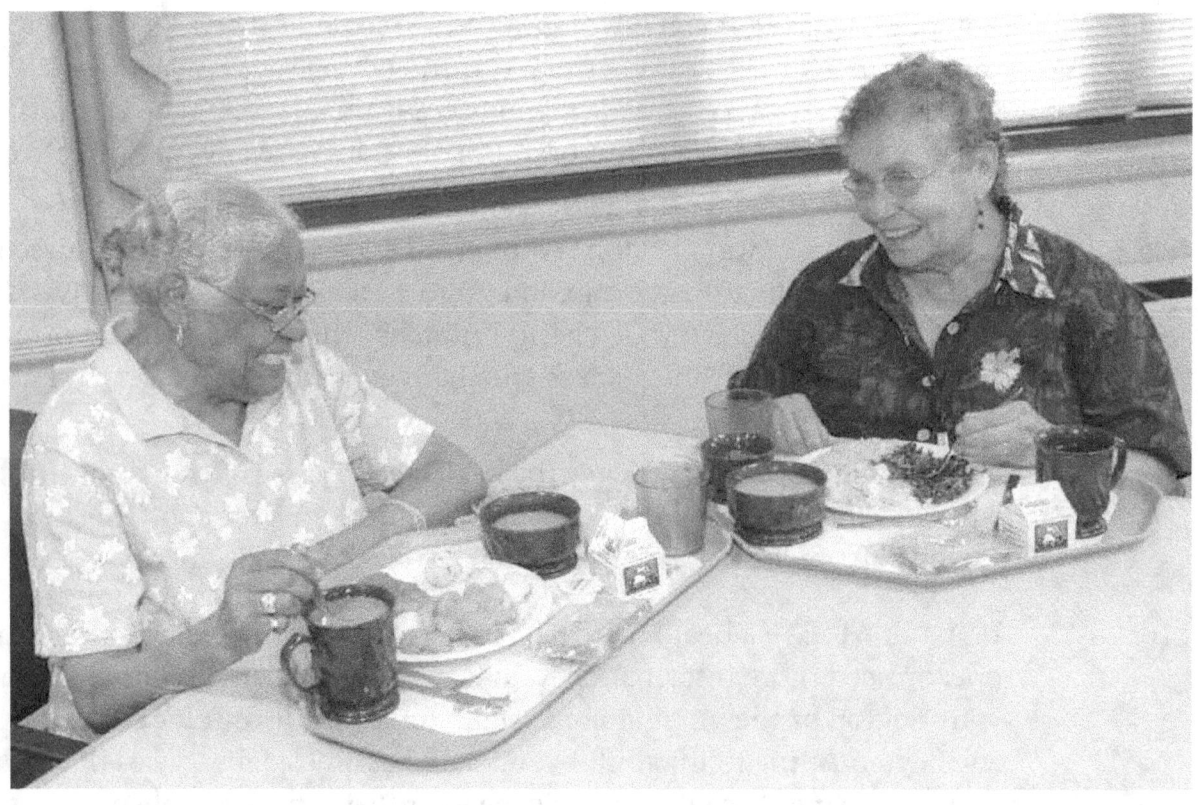

Paying for Nursing Home Care and Other Health Care Costs

4

Overview

Nursing home care can be very expensive. There are many ways you can pay for nursing home care. For example, you can use your own money, you may be able to get help from your state, or you may use long-term care insurance.

Most people who enter nursing homes begin by paying for their care out of their own pocket. As you use your resources (like bank accounts, stocks, etc.) over a period of time, you may eventually become eligible for Medicaid.

If you have Medicare and need nursing home care

Medicare generally **doesn't** cover long-term stays (room and board) in a nursing home. Also, nursing home care isn't covered by many types of health insurance. However, don't drop your health care coverage (including Medicare) if you're in a nursing home. Even if it doesn't cover nursing home care, you will need health coverage for hospital care, doctor services, and medical supplies while you're in the nursing home.

Medicare covers skilled nursing facility (SNF) care in a Medicare-certified skilled nursing facility for a limited time after a 3-day qualifying hospital stay. For more information on Medicare coverage of skilled nursing facility care, get a free copy of the booklet "Medicare Coverage of Skilled Nursing Facility Care." See page 59.

This section explains some of the ways you can pay for a long-term stay in a nursing home, or get help with other health care costs. It includes information about the following:

- Personal resources (see page 42)
- Help from your state—Medicaid (see pages 42–44)
- Long-term care insurance (see page 45)
- Coming soon—The Community Living Assistance Services and Supports (CLASS) Program (see page 46)
- Medicare (see page 46–49)

Words in blue are defined on pages 67–68.

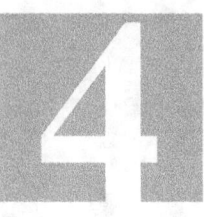

Personal resources

You can use your personal money and savings to pay for nursing home care. Some insurance companies let you use your life insurance policy to pay for long-term care. Ask your insurance agent how this works.

Important: Be sure to get help before using either of these options. There are important issues you need to understand.

Help from your state (Medicaid)

Medicaid pays for care for about 7 out of every 10 nursing home residents. Medicaid is a joint state and Federal program that pays for certain health services and nursing home care for older people with limited income and resources. If you qualify, you may be able to get help to pay for nursing home care or other health care costs. If you qualify for both Medicare and Medicaid, most health care costs are covered. But remember not all nursing homes accept Medicaid payment.

Check with the nursing home to see if they accept people with Medicaid, and if they have a Medicaid bed available. Who is eligible for Medicaid and what services are covered varies from state to state. Most often, eligibility is based on your income and personal resources. You may be eligible for Medicaid coverage in a nursing home even if you haven't qualified for other Medicaid services in the past.

Sometimes you won't be eligible until you have spent some of your personal resources on medical care. You may be moved to another room in the Medicaid-certified section of the nursing home when your care is paid by Medicaid. To get more information on Medicaid eligibility requirements in your state, call your State Medical Assistance (Medicaid) office. See pages 63–65.

Words in blue are defined on pages 67–68.

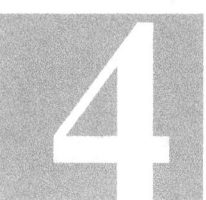

Paying for Nursing Home Care and Other Health Care Costs

Some important things to know about Medicaid

- **Your home:** The state can't put a lien on your home if there is a reasonable chance you'll return home after getting nursing home care or if you have a spouse or dependents living there. This means they can't take, sell, or hold your property to recover benefits that are correctly paid for nursing home care while you're living in a nursing home in this circumstance.

  In most cases, after a person who gets Medicaid nursing home benefits passes away, the state must try to get whatever benefits it paid for that person back from their estate. However, they can't recover on a lien against the person's home if it's the residence of the person's spouse, sibling (who has an equity interest and was residing in the home at least one year prior to the nursing home admission), or a blind or disabled child or a child under the age of 21 in the family.

- **Your assets:** Most people who are eligible for Medicaid have to reduce their assets first. There are rules about what's counted as an asset and what isn't when determining Medicaid eligibility. There are also rules that require states to allow married couples to protect a certain amount of assets and income when one of them is in an institution (like a nursing home) and one isn't.

  A spouse who isn't in an institution may keep one half of the couples' joint assets, up to a maximum of $109,560 in 2011, as well as a monthly income allowance. For more information, call your State Medical Assistance (Medicaid) office. See pages 63–65. You can also call your local Area Agency on Aging to find out if your state has any legal services where you could get more information. You can also get free health insurance counseling from your State Health Insurance Assistance Program (SHIP). See pages 63–65.

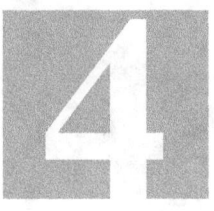

Some important things to know about Medicaid (continued)

- **Transferring your assets:** You can't give your assets away to family members or non-family members, rather than use your assets to pay for your nursing home care. If you give assets away within 5 years before the date you apply for Medicaid, or even after you apply, the gift may be treated as a transfer of assets for less than fair market value.

Transfers for less than fair market value may subject you to a penalty, and the penalty is that Medicaid won't pay for your nursing home care for a period of time. How long that period is depends on the value of the assets you gave away. There are limited exceptions to this, especially if you have a spouse, or a blind or disabled child. But as a general rule, giving away your assets can result in no payment for your nursing home care, possibly for many months or even years.

Note: Federal law protects spouses of nursing home residents from losing all of their income and assets to pay for nursing home care for their spouse. When one member of a couple enters a nursing home and applies for Medicaid, his or her eligibility is determined under "spousal impoverishment" rules.

Spousal impoverishment helps make sure that the spouse still at home will have the money needed to pay for living expenses by protecting a certain amount of the couple's resources, as well as at least a portion of the nursing home resident's income, for the use of the spouse who is still at home. For more information about this protection, call your State Medical Assistance (Medicaid) office. See pages 63–65.

To apply for Medicaid, call your State Medical Assistance (Medicaid) office. See pages 63–65. They can tell you if you qualify for the Medicaid nursing home benefit or other programs, such as the Programs of All-Inclusive Care for the Elderly (PACE), or home and community-based waiver programs. See page 14.

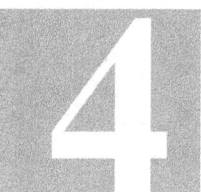

Long-term care insurance

This type of private insurance policy can help pay for many types of long-term care, including both skilled and nonskilled (custodial) care. Long-term care insurance can vary widely. Some policies may cover only nursing home care. Others may include coverage for a whole range of services like adult day care, assisted living, medical equipment, and informal home care.

If you have long-term care insurance, check your policy or call the insurance company to find out if the care you need is covered. If you're shopping for long-term care insurance, find out which types of long-term care services and facilities the different policies cover. Also, check to see if your coverage could be limited because of a pre-existing condition. Make sure you buy from a reliable company that is licensed in your state.

For more information about long-term care insurance, get a copy of "A Shopper's Guide to Long-Term Care Insurance" from the National Association of Insurance Commissioners, by visiting www.naic.org/index_ltc_section.htm.

Federal employees, members of the Uniformed Services, retirees, their spouses, and other qualified relatives may be able to buy long-term care insurance at discounted group rates. For more information about long-term care insurance for Federal employees, visit www.opm.gov/insure/ltc.

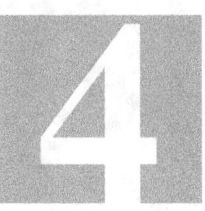

New—The Community Living Assistance Services and Supports (CLASS) Program

The CLASS Program will be a national, voluntary insurance program to help pay for services and supports needed to live as independently as possible. CLASS is not yet available. Eligible working adults will be able to enroll in the CLASS program when it begins. Following a 5-year vesting period, enrollees who meet certain eligibility requirements (such as needing assistance with activities of daily living) will have access to the benefit. Visit www.healthcare.gov to learn more.

Medicare for your health care and prescription drugs

Medicare

Medicare is a health insurance program for people age 65 or older, under age 65 with certain disabilities, and any age with End-Stage Renal Disease (ESRD) (permanent kidney failure requiring dialysis or a kidney transplant).

People get Medicare health care in two ways:

1. **Original Medicare**

   Original Medicare **doesn't** pay for most nursing home care. Most nursing home care is custodial care to help with activities of daily living like bathing, dressing, and using the bathroom. Medicare covers very limited and medically-necessary skilled care or home health care if you need skilled care for an illness or injury and you meet certain conditions.

   For more information on Medicare coverage of skilled nursing facility (SNF) care or home health care, visit www.medicare.gov/Publications to view or print a copy of the booklet "Medicare Coverage of Skilled Nursing Facility Care" or "Medicare and Home Health Care." You can also order a free copy by calling 1-800-MEDICARE (1-800-633-4227). TTY users should call 1-877-486-2048.

4

Medicare for your health care and prescription drugs (continued)

2. **Medicare Advantage Plans and Other Medicare Health Plans**

   If you belong to a Medicare Advantage Plan (Part C) (like an HMO or PPO) or other Medicare health plan, check with your plan to see if it covers nursing home care. Usually, plans **don't** help pay for this care unless the nursing home has a contract with the plan. Ask the health plan about nursing home coverage before you make any arrangements. If the nursing home has a contract with your health plan, ask the health plan if they check the home for quality of care.

Medicare Prescription Drug Coverage (Part D)

If you belong to a Medicare Prescription Drug Plan and live in a nursing home or other institution, you'll get your covered prescriptions from a long-term care pharmacy that works with your plan. (**Note:** Institutions don't include assisted living or adult living facilities or residential homes, or any kind of nursing home not identified by Medicare.) This long-term care pharmacy usually contracts with (or is owned and operated by) your institution.

Words in blue are defined on pages 67–68.

Unless someone chooses a Medicare health plan with drug coverage or a stand-alone Medicare Prescription Drug Plan, Medicare automatically enrolls people with both Medicare and full Medicaid coverage living in institutions into Medicare Prescription Drug Plans. If you live in a nursing home and have full Medicaid coverage, you pay nothing for your covered prescriptions after Medicaid has paid for your stay for at least 1 full calendar month.

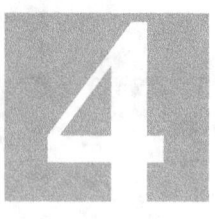

If you have Medicare and live in a nursing home or other institution, you should also know the following:

- If you move into or move out of a nursing home or other institution, you can switch Medicare drug plans at that time. You can switch Medicare drug plans at any time while you're living in the institution.

- If you aren't able to join on your own, your authorized representative can enroll you in a plan that meets your needs.

- If you're in a skilled nursing facility getting Medicare-covered skilled nursing care, your prescriptions generally will be covered by Medicare Part A (Hospital Insurance).

Hospital stays and Skilled Nursing Facility Care

If you have Original Medicare or a Medicare health plan, you should also know the following:

- **If you need short-term care in a Skilled Nursing Facility after a Medicare-covered inpatient hospital stay of 3 days or more**, the hospital staff should help you find a Medicare-certified facility that gives the skilled care you need. For more information on Medicare coverage of skilled nursing facility care, view the booklet "Medicare Coverage of Skilled Nursing Facility Care." See page 59.

- **If you think you're being asked to leave a hospital (discharged) too soon**, you can ask for a review from your Quality Improvement Organization (QIO). The QIO is an independent reviewer who will give you a second opinion about whether you're ready to leave the hospital. Your hospital services will continue to be paid during the review (except for charges like your coinsurance and deductibles). Visit www.medicare.gov/contacts or call 1-800-MEDICARE (1-800-633-4227) for the QIO's phone number. TTY users should call 1-877-486-2048.

- **If you think you're being asked to leave a skilled nursing facility too soon**, you can ask for a review from your QIO. The QIO, under most circumstances, will give you its decision before Medicare coverage of your skilled nursing care ends. For the QIO's phone number, visit www.medicare.gov/contacts or call 1-800-MEDICARE.

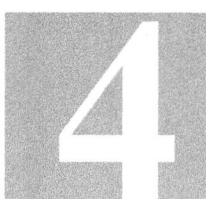

Hospital stays and Skilled Nursing Facility Care (continued)

For anyone being discharged from a health care setting like a hospital or skilled nursing facility: Use Medicare's "Your Discharge Planning Checklist" to help make sure you have all the information you need before you're discharged. To get a copy, see page 59.

Get your personalized Medicare information

Register at www.MyMedicare.gov, Medicare's secure online service for accessing your personal Medicare information.

- Create and print an "On the Go" report that lists information you can share with your providers.

- Add or modify self-reported health management information, such as medical conditions and allergies.

- View or modify your personal drug list and pharmacy information, and see your prescription drug costs.

- Search for and create a list of your favorite providers, and access quality information about them.

- Complete your Initial Enrollment Questionnaire so your bills can get paid correctly.

- Track your Original Medicare claims, and order a Medicare Summary Notice.

- Check your Part B deductible status.

- View your eligibility information.

- Get notices about what services you will be eligible for in the coming year.

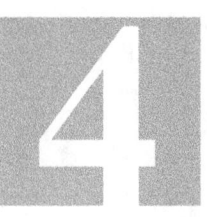

Paying for Nursing Home Care and Other Health Care Costs

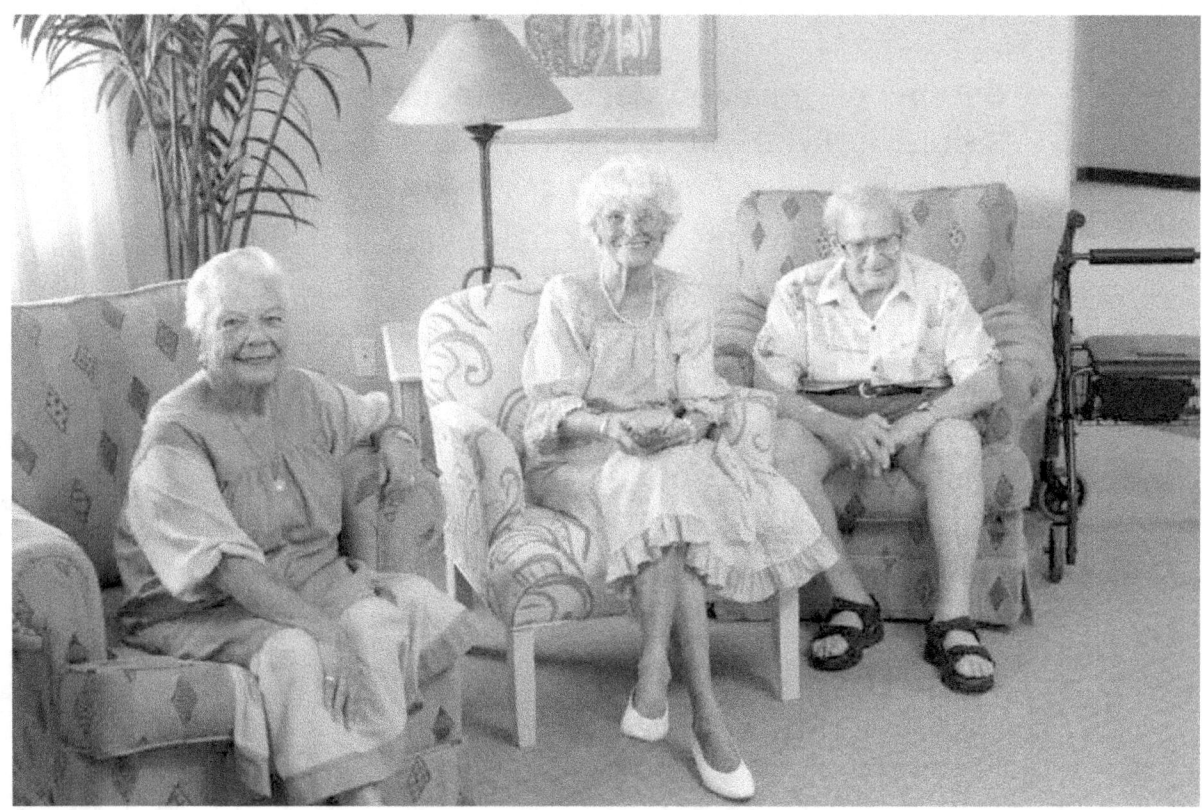

Care plans

The nursing home staff will get your health information and review your health condition to prepare your care plan. You (if you're able), your family (with your permission), or someone acting on your behalf has the right to take part in planning your care with the nursing home staff.

Your care plan is very important. A good care plan can help make sure that you're getting the care you need and help make your stay more pleasant. Your health assessment (a review of your health condition) begins on the day you're admitted. A comprehensive assessment must be completed within 14 days of admission. You should expect to get a health assessment at least every 90 days after your first review, and possibly more often if your medical status changes.

The nursing home staff will assess your condition regularly to see if your health status has changed. They will adjust your care plan as needed. Nursing homes are required to submit this information to the federal government. This information is used for quality measures, nursing home payment, and state inspections.

Depending on your needs, your care plan may include the following:

- What kind of personal or health care services you need
- What type of staff should give you these services
- How often you need the services
- What kind of equipment or supplies you need (like a wheelchair or feeding tube)
- What kind of diet you need (if you need a special one)
- Your health goal (or goals)
- How your care plan will help you reach your goals

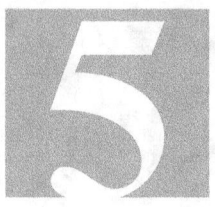

Reporting and resolving problems

If you have a problem at the nursing home, talk to the staff involved. For example, if you have a problem with your care, talk to the nurse or Certified Nurse Assistant (CNA). The staff may not know there is a problem unless you tell them. If the problem isn't resolved, ask to talk with the supervisor, social worker, director of nursing, administrator, or your doctor.

Words in blue are defined on pages 67–68.

The Medicare and/or Medicaid-certified nursing home must have a grievance procedure for complaints. If your problem isn't resolved, follow the facility's grievance procedure. You may also want to bring the problem to the resident or family council.

A Medicare and/or Medicaid-certified nursing home must post the name, address, and phone number of state groups, such as the State Survey Agency, State Licensure Office, State Ombudsman Program, Protection and Advocacy Network, and the Medicaid Fraud Control Unit. If you feel you need outside help to resolve your problem, call the Long-Term Care Ombudsman or State Survey Agency for your area. See pages 63–65.

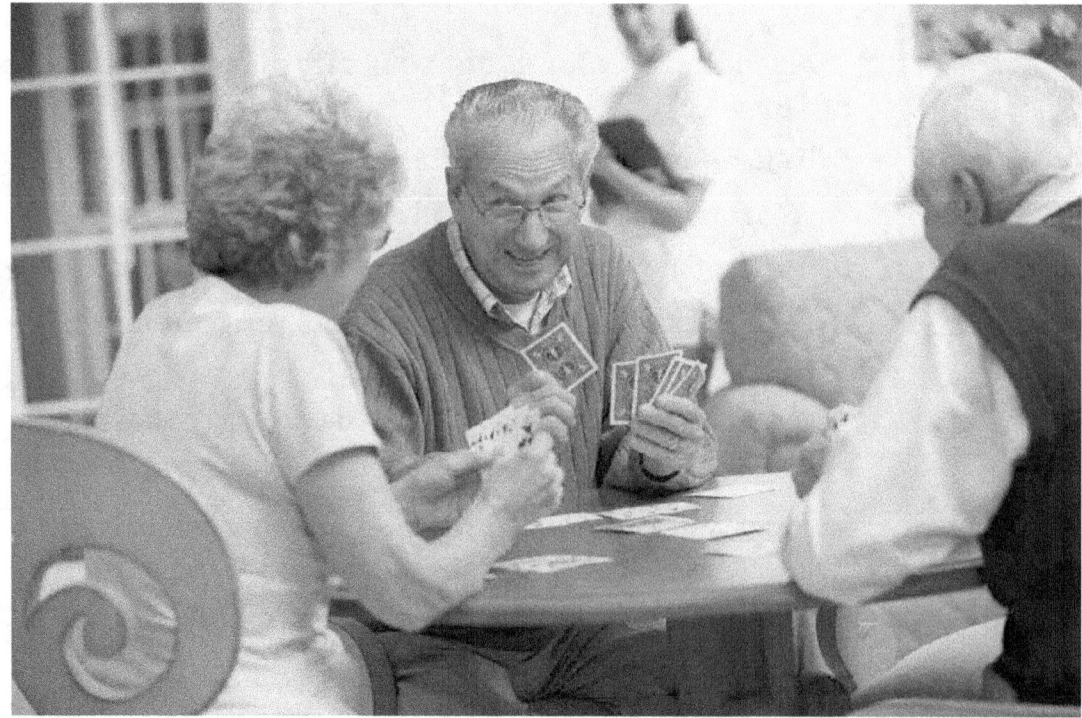

5

Your resident rights and protections

What are my rights in Medicare and/or Medicaid-certified nursing homes?

As a resident in a Medicare and/or Medicaid-certified nursing home, you have certain rights and protections under Federal and state law that help ensure you get the care and services you need. You have the right to be informed, make your own decisions, and have your personal information kept private.

The nursing home must tell you about these rights and explain them in writing in a language you understand. They must also explain in writing how you should act and what you're responsible for while you're in the nursing home. This must be done before or at the time you're admitted, as well as during your stay. You must acknowledge in writing that you got this information.

At a minimum, Federal law specifies that a nursing home must protect and promote the following rights of each resident:

- **Be treated with respect:** You have the right to be treated with dignity and respect, as well as make your own schedule and participate in the activities you choose. You have the right to decide when you go to bed, rise in the morning, and eat your meals.

- **Participate in activities:** You have the right to participate in an activities program designed to meet your needs and the needs of the other residents.

- **Be free from discrimination:** Nursing homes don't have to accept all applicants, but they must comply with local, state, and Federal civil rights laws. If you believe you have been discriminated against, call the Department of Health and Human Services, Office for Civil Rights at 1-800-368-1019 or visit www.hhs.gov/ocr. TTY users should call 1-800-537-7697.

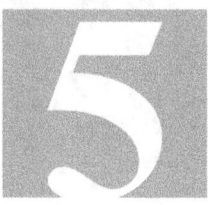

Your resident rights and protections (continued)

- **Be free from abuse and neglect:** You have the right to be free from verbal, sexual, physical, and mental abuse. Nursing homes can't keep you apart from everyone else against your will. If you feel you have been mistreated (abused) or the nursing home isn't meeting your needs (neglect), report this to the nursing home, your family, your local Long-Term Care Ombudsman, or State Survey Agency. The nursing home must investigate and report all suspected violations and any injuries of unknown origin within 5 working days of the incident to the proper authorities.

- **Be free from restraints:** Nursing homes can't use any physical restraints (like side rails) or chemical restraints (like drugs) to discipline you for the staff's own convenience.

- **Make complaints:** You have the right to make a complaint to the staff of the nursing home or any other person without fear of being punished. The nursing home must address the issue promptly.

- **Get proper medical care:** You have the following rights regarding your medical care:
  - To be fully informed about your total health status in a language you understand.
  - To be fully informed about your medical condition, prescription and over-the-counter drugs, vitamins, and supplements.
  - To be involved in the choice of your doctor.
  - To participate in the decisions that affect your care.
  - To take part in developing your care plan. By law, nursing homes must develop a care plan for each resident. You have the right to take part in this process. Family members can also help with your care plan with your permission.
  - To access all your records and reports, including clinical records (medical records and reports) promptly during weekdays. Your legal guardian has the right to look at all your medical records and make important decisions on your behalf.
  - To express any complaints (also called "grievances") you have about your care or treatment.
  - To create advance directives (a health care proxy or power of attorney, a living will, or after-death wishes) in accordance with State law.
  - To refuse to participate in experimental treatment.

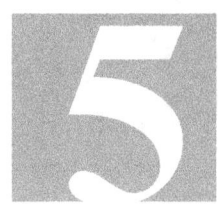

- **Have your representative notified:** The nursing home must notify your doctor and, if known, your legal representative or an interested family member when the following occurs:

  — You're injured in an accident and/or need to see a doctor.

  — Your physical, mental, or psychosocial status starts to get worse.

  — You have a life threatening condition.

  — You have medical complications.

  — Your treatment needs to change significantly.

  — The nursing home decides to transfer or discharge you from the nursing home.

- **Get information on services and fees:** You have the right to be told in writing about all nursing home services and fees (those that are charged and not charged to you) before you move into the nursing home and at any time when services and fees change. In addition:

  — The nursing home can't require a minimum entrance fee if your care is paid for by Medicare or Medicaid.

  — For people seeking admission to the nursing home, the nursing home must tell you (both orally and in writing) and display written information about how to apply for and use Medicare and Medicaid benefits.

  — The nursing home must also provide information on how to get a refund if you paid for an item or service, but because of Medicare and Medicaid eligibility rules, it's now considered covered.

Your resident rights and protections (continued)

- **Manage your money:** You have the right to manage your own money or choose someone you trust to do this for you. In addition:

  — If you deposit your money with the nursing home or ask them to hold or account for your money, you must sign a written statement saying you want them to do this.

  — The nursing home must allow you access to your bank accounts, cash, and other financial records.

  — The nursing home must have a system that ensures full accounting for your funds and can't combine your funds with the nursing home's funds.

  — The nursing home must protect your funds from any loss by providing an acceptable protection, such as buying a surety bond.

  — If a resident with a fund passes away, the nursing home must return the funds with a final accounting to the person or court handling the resident's estate within 30 days.

- **Get proper privacy, property, and living arrangements:** You have the following rights:

  — To keep and use your personal belongings and property as long as they don't interfere with the rights, health, or safety of others.

  — To have private visits.

  — To make and get private phone calls.

  — To have privacy in sending and getting mail and email.

  — To have the nursing home protect your property from theft.

  — To share a room with your spouse if you both live in the same nursing home (if you both agree to do so).

  — The nursing home has to notify you before your room or your roommate is changed and should take your preferences into account.

  — To review the nursing home's health and fire safety inspection results.

- **Spend time with visitors:** You have the following rights:
  — To spend private time with visitors.

  — To have visitors at any time, as long as you wish to see them, and as long as the visit doesn't interfere with the provision of care and privacy rights of other residents.

  — To see any person who gives you help with your health, social, legal, or other services at any time. This includes your doctor, a representative from the health department, and your Long-Term Care Ombudsman, among others.

- **Get social services:** The nursing home must provide you with any needed social services, including the following:
  — Counseling

  — Help solving problems with other residents

  — Help in contacting legal and financial professionals

  — Discharge planning

- **Leave the nursing home:**
  — **Leaving for visits:** If your health allows, and your doctor agrees, you can spend time away from the nursing home visiting family or friends during the day or overnight, called a "leave of absence." Talk to the nursing home staff a few days ahead of time so the staff has time to prepare your medicines and write your instructions.
  Caution: If your nursing home care is covered by certain health insurance, you may not be able to leave for visits without losing your coverage.

  — **Moving out:** Living in a nursing home is your choice. You can choose to move to another place. However, the nursing home may have a policy that requires you to tell them before you plan to leave. If you don't, you may have to pay an extra fee.

Your resident rights and protections (continued)

- **Have protections against unfair transfer or discharge:** You can't be sent to another nursing home or made to leave the nursing home, unless any of the following are true:

  — It's necessary for the welfare, health, or safety of you or others.

  — Your health has improved to the point that nursing home care is no longer necessary.

  — The nursing home hasn't been paid for services you got.

  — The nursing home closes.

  You have the following rights:

  — You have the right to appeal a transfer or discharge to the State Survey Agency. See pages 63–65 for the phone number for your state.

  — The nursing home can't make you leave if you're waiting to get Medicaid.

  — Except in emergencies, nursing homes must give a 30-day written notice of their plan and reason to discharge or transfer you.

  — The nursing home has to safely and orderly transfer or discharge you and give you proper notice of bed-hold and readmission requirements.

- **Form or participate in resident groups:** You have a right to form or participate in a resident group to discuss issues and concerns about the nursing home's policies and operations. Most homes have such groups, often called "resident councils." The home must give you meeting space and must listen to and act upon grievances and recommendations of the group.

- **Have your family and friends involved:** Family and friends can help make sure you get good quality care. They can visit and get to know the staff and the nursing home's rules. Family members and legal guardians may meet with the families of other residents and may participate in family councils, if one exists. With your permission, family members can help with your care plan. If a family member or friend is your legal guardian, he or she has the right to look at all medical records about you and make important decisions on your behalf.

Free booklets on Medicare, Medicaid, and related topics

To read, print, or order free booklets on Medicare and related topics, including those listed below, visit www.medicare.gov/Publications. You may also be able to order a free copy by calling 1-800-MEDICARE (1-800-633-4227). Some booklets are available in Spanish, Braille, Large Print (English and Spanish), and on audio-cassette. TTY users should call 1-877-486-2048.

- "Medicare & You"—This handbook gives basic information about Medicare coverage and benefits, health plan choices, rights and protections, and more.

- "If You Need Help Paying Medicare Costs, There Are Programs That Can Help You"—This brochure has information about Medicare Savings Programs that can help you pay health care costs.

- "Medicare Coverage of Skilled Nursing Facility Care"—This booklet explains when and how much Medicare covers for skilled nursing facility care.

- "Medicare and Home Health Care"—This booklet explains Medicare coverage of home health care.

- "Medicare Hospice Benefits"—This booklet explains Medicare coverage of hospice care for people who have a terminal illness.

- "Your Guide to Medicare Prescription Drug Coverage"—This booklet explains how Medicare prescription drug coverage works, how this coverage may affect your current drug coverage, and how to get Extra Help if you have limited income or resources.

- "Your Discharge Planning Checklist"—This checklist lists important information for patients and caregivers who are preparing to leave a hospital, nursing home, or other health care setting.

- "Your Right to Get Information About Returning to the Community"—This brochure gives contact information for nursing home residents who want to find out more about leaving a nursing home and getting all the services and support they need to live in the community.

Words in blue are defined on pages 67–68.

For More Information

To get help with questions about Medicare

Call 1-800-MEDICARE (1-800-633-4227). TTY users should call 1-877-486-2048. If you need help in a language other than English, tell the customer services representative.

For information on specific questions and diseases

You or someone you care for may need nursing home care because of a specific physical or mental health condition. It may be helpful for you to understand the health condition. This will help you plan for future health and personal care needs. The organizations below can answer your questions about specific health conditions and diseases.

Organization	Phone	Web Site
Alzheimer's Disease		
Alzheimer's Association 225 N. Michigan Avenue Floor 17 Chicago, Illinois 60601-7652	1-800-272-3900	www.alz.org
Arthritis		
Arthritis Foundation P.O. Box 7669 Atlanta, Georgia 30357-0669	1-800-568-4045	www.arthritis.org
Cancer		
American Cancer Society 1599 Clifton Road Atlanta, Georgia 30329	1-800-227-2345	www.cancer.org
National Cancer Institute (NCI) Public Inquiries Office Room 10A O331 Center Drive MSC 2580 Bethesda, Maryland 20892-2580	1-800-422-6237 TTY: 1-800-332-8615	www.cancer.gov

Organization	Phone	Web Site
Diabetes		
American Diabetes Association Attn: National Call Center 1701 N. Beauregard Street Alexandria, Virginia 22311	1-800-342-2383	www.diabetes.org
Heart Disease		
American Heart Association National Center 7272 Greenville Avenue Dallas, Texas 75231	1-800-242-8721 Call for local address.	www.heart.org
Kidney Disease		
American Kidney Fund 6110 Executive Boulevard Suite 1010 Rockville, Maryland 20852	1-800-638-8299	www.kidneyfund.org
National Kidney and Urologic Diseases Information Clearinghouse 3 Information Way Bethesda, Maryland 20892-3580	1-800-891-5390	www.kidney.niddk.nih.gov
National Kidney Foundation 30 E. 33rd Street New York, New York 10016	1-800-622-9010	www.kidney.org
Mental Health		
National Institute of Mental Health Public Information and Communication Branch 6001 Executive Boulevard Room 8184, MSC 9663 Bethesda, Maryland 20892-9663	1-866-615-6464 TTY: 1-866-415-8051	www.nimh.nih.gov

For More Information

Information about specific conditions and diseases (continued)

Organization	Phone	Web Site
Multiple Sclerosis		
National Multiple Sclerosis Society 733 Third Avenue New York, New York 10017	1-800-FIGHT-MS (1-800-344-4867)	www.nmss.org
Osteoporosis		
National Osteoporosis Foundation 1232 22nd Street NW Washington, DC 20037-1292	1-800-231-4222	www.nof.org
Parkinson Disease		
National Parkinson Foundation 1501 NW 9th Avenue/Bob Hope Road Miami, Florida 33136-1494	1-800-227-2345	www.parkinson.org
Stroke		
National Stroke Association 9707 E. Easter Lane Englewood, Colorado 80112	1-800-422-6237 TTY: 1-800-332-8615	www.stroke.org

This page has been intentionally left blank.
The printed version contains phone number
information. For the most recent phone
number information, please visit
www.medicare.gov/contacts or call
1-800-MEDICARE (1-800-633-4227).
TTY users should call 1-877-486-2048.
Thank you.

6

For More Information

This page has been intentionally left blank. The printed version contains phone number information. For the most recent phone number information, please visit www.medicare.gov/contacts or call 1-800-MEDICARE (1-800-633-4227). TTY users should call 1-877-486-2048. Thank you.

This page has been intentionally left blank.
The printed version contains phone number
information. For the most recent phone
number information, please visit
www.medicare.gov/contacts or call
1-800-MEDICARE (1-800-633-4227).
TTY users should call 1-877-486-2048.
Thank you.

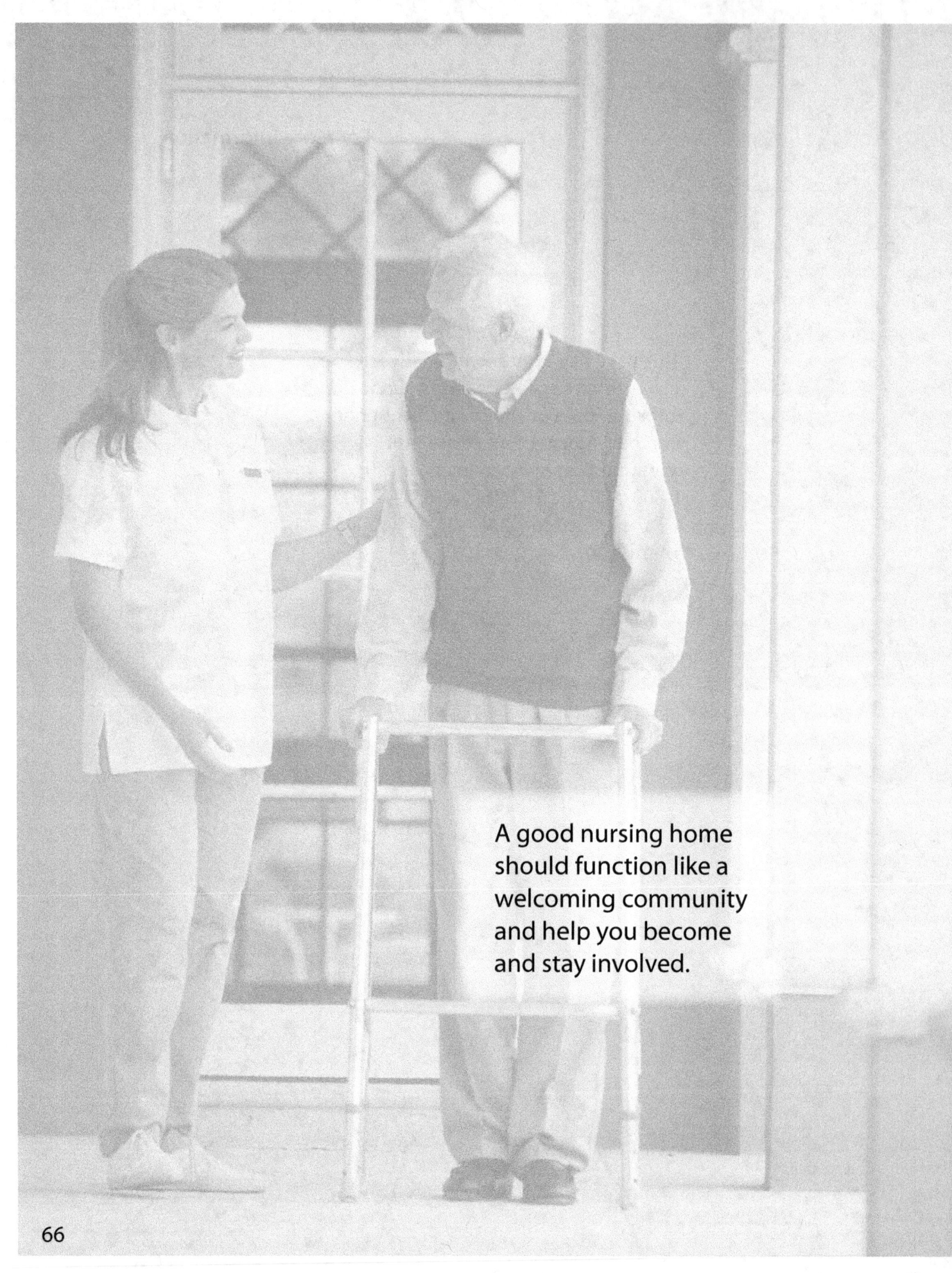

A good nursing home should function like a welcoming community and help you become and stay involved.

Custodial Care—Nonskilled personal care, such as help with activities of daily living like bathing, dressing, eating, getting in or out of a bed or chair, moving around, and using the bathroom. It may also include the kind of health-related care that most people do themselves, like using eye drops. In most cases, Medicare doesn't pay for custodial care.

End-Stage Renal Disease (ESRD)—Permanent kidney failure that requires a regular course of dialysis or a kidney transplant.

Long-Term Care Ombudsman—An independent advocate (supporter) for nursing home and assisted living facility residents who works to solve problems between residents and nursing homes or assisted living facilities. They may be able to provide information about home health agencies in their area.

Medicaid—A joint Federal and state program that helps with medical costs for some people with limited income and resources. Medicaid programs vary from state to state, but most health care costs are covered if you qualify for both Medicare and Medicaid.

Medicare—The Federal health insurance program for people who are age 65 or older, certain younger people with disabilities, and people with End-Stage Renal Disease (permanent kidney failure requiring dialysis or a transplant, sometimes called ESRD).

Medicare Advantage Plan (Part C)—A type of Medicare health plan offered by a private company that contracts with Medicare to provide you with all your Medicare Part A and Part B benefits. Medicare Advantage Plans include Health Maintenance Organizations, Preferred Provider Organizations, Private Fee-for-Service Plans, Special Needs Plans, and Medicare Medical Savings Account Plans. If you're enrolled in a Medicare Advantage Plan, Medicare services are covered through the plan and aren't paid for under Original Medicare. Most Medicare Advantage Plans offer prescription drug coverage.

Medicare Health Plan—A Medicare health plan is offered by a private company that contracts with Medicare to provide Part A and Part B benefits to people with Medicare who enroll in the plan.

Medicare Prescription Drug Plan (Part D)—A stand-alone drug plan that adds prescription drug coverage to Original Medicare, some Medicare Cost Plans, some Medicare Private-Fee-for-Service Plans, and Medicare Medical Savings Account Plans. These plans are offered by insurance companies and other private companies approved by Medicare. Medicare Advantage Plans may also offer prescription drug coverage that follows the same rules as Medicare Prescription Drug Plans.

Original Medicare—Original Medicare is fee-for-service coverage under which the government pays your health care providers directly for your Part A and/or Part B benefits.

Skilled Nursing Facility (SNF)—A nursing facility with the staff and equipment to give skilled nursing care and, in most cases, skilled rehabilitative services and other related health services.

Skilled Nursing Facility Care—Skilled nursing care and rehabilitation services provided on a continuous, daily basis, in a skilled nursing facility. Examples of skilled nursing facility care include physical therapy or intravenous injections that can only be given by a registered nurse or doctor.

State Health Insurance Assistance Program (SHIP)—A state program that gets money from the Federal government to give free local health insurance counseling to people with Medicare.

State Medical Assistance (Medicaid) Office—A state agency that is in charge of the state's Medicaid program and can give information about programs to help pay medical bills for people with limited income and resources.

State Survey Agency—A state agency that oversees health care facilities that participate in the Medicare and/or Medicaid programs. The State Survey Agency inspects health care facilities and investigates complaints to ensure that health and safety standards are met.

8 Index

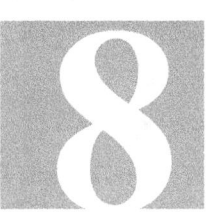

**U.S. DEPARTMENT OF HEALTH
AND HUMAN SERVICES**

Centers for Medicare & Medicaid Services
7500 Security Boulevard
Baltimore, Maryland 21244-1850

Official Business
Penalty for Private Use, $300

CMS Product No. 02174
Revised May 2011

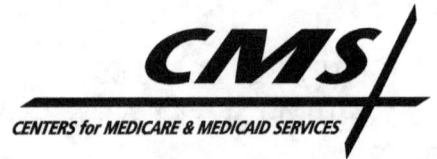

This booklet is available in Spanish. To get a free
copy, call 1-800-MEDICARE (1-800-633-4227).
TTY users should call 1-877-486-2048.

¿Necesita usted una copia en español?
Para obtener su copia GRATIS, llame al
1-800-MEDICARE (1-800-633-4227).

For more information about nursing homes,
visit www.medicare.gov/NHCompare.